Cure Your Sex Addic

MW01243810

TABLE OF CONTENTS

CHAPTER 1

THE HISTORICAL BACKGROUND

As with all addictions, addiction to sex starts in small ways and gradually creeps more and more into one's life. Like a train with no brakes, the progress of this problem is hard to stop once in motion. The desire can swiftly turn into need, the need into craving and the craving into a desperate chasm of desire that can never be filled.

Finally there is a realisation that the craving for sex has taken over and one is powerless to escape. You may come to the shocking realisation that sex has control over you and not the other way round. Then in addition to the addictive behaviour there grows a toxic sense of shame and failure.

Sex is a normal human activity, so how come it can turn into a problem? It's how we show love to each other; It's fun to do; it is relaxing; we need to do it to reproduce; it's natural, so what's the problem? In order to answer this fully, I need to explore healthy attitudes to sex and compare them with unhealthy ones. In order to do this I'm going to put our attitude towards sex into some historical context so we can make some valid comparisons.

I'm going to start by describing a recent time when society was more stable and people were generally happier. Thanks to the stability of families, there were less social problems to cause stress and mental illness. There were lower rates of family breakdown and linked problems that can traumatise children and create damaged adults. It is the underlying premise of this book that when one is emotionally damaged, this opens the door for addictive behaviour.

Sex is just one of the things that people become addicted to when they are unhappy, lonely, feeling rejected, sad and unlovable.

We live in a an 'over sexed era' where sex has been paraded in front of us in the media as entertainment and used to sell commodities. Sex has been cheapened and has been made into a marketable commodity in its own right. However it may come as a surprise to the reader that prior to this era, there were much stricter taboos across society about who could have sex and when. Censorship ensured that films, books, television and radio programmes adhered to a strict code of decency and there were strict limits on what could be broadcast. People were also much more religious and this strongly affected the way they behaved and their attitudes to sex.

Prior to 1970 the age of majority was 21. This means that all young people were still considered to be the responsibility of their parents until they reached the age of 21. The practical upshot of this was that kids stayed at home for much longer and weren't thrown out of the house until they'd had time to mature. Living with mum and dad has a very steadying effect on older teenagers and would have had a decided effect on when they became sexually active.

There were very strict taboos against sex before marriage. One was expected to go courting, get engaged and then later get married, and then and only then become sexually active. Getting pregnant before marriage was very much frowned upon.

In my formative years, the 1950s and 1960s, it would have been perfectly correct to describe the UK as a Christian country. In fact Britain has been a Christian country since the first or second century under the Roman 'Emperor Tiberius. Later the Emperor Constantine decreed that the whole of the Roman empire would follow Christianity. It had a further boost in the 6th Century when Celtic Christianity was brought by monks to the mainland from Ireland. It was rapidly adopted as the main faith and has shaped the way the British have thought and acted ever since. It is hard to overemphasize the importance that Christianity has had on shaping the British culture and character, being the founder of the education system, the legal system and many other British institutions.

In the 1950s, the church's moral code still had a huge of influence on the behaviour of most people in society. The majority of schools were afiliated to the Church and so at the beginning of every single school day there would have been a religious assembly. Because of this religious connection with the upbringing and education of children, there were far stronger morality teachings in schools. As a result, children were far less 'sexualized' and childhood lasted longer. Children remained innocent for longer and became sexually active much later in their lives.

This all helped to reinforce the general consensus that sex was something that should only take place between married couples. In fact people didn't even talk about sex openly like they do these days. It was considered to be a topic far too intimate and risky that adults should only discuss in the privacy of their bedrooms, and certainly never in public or with their children. Discussing such topics on the television or internet just didn't happen. Portraying the sexual act on film and television wasn't allowed due the strict censorship that existed prior to the 1970s.

The overwhelming opinion of society was that sex was an activity that should only occur in the context of a committed married relationship. Moreover, there was an implicit agreement that any resulting children would be given a stable upbringing by both parents. Divorce was frowned on by society and for this reason there was a huge social stigma around it. People were more conscious of their personal responsibility for taking care of their own children and the elderly, since the Welfare State hadn't yet grown into the gargantuan and extremely expensive structure that it has become.

Roles within the family were very narrowly defined. After the 2nd World War it was pretty much universally agreed that the mother would stay at home and look after the children until they finished secondary education. The father was expected to be the bread winner and it was his role to protect and provide for his children until they were 'launched'. The result of this was that children generally grew up in an atmosphere of peace and security.

There used to be far less geographic mobility amongst the population. Ownership of cars was rare in the period of post war austerity. Children tended to live their adult lives in or close to the same area as their parents, enabling families to stay in much more in contact. The 'extended family' was always there to give support resulting in far less social isolation and a greater degree of security. This also contributed to a lower incidence of social anxiety and mental health issues caused by loneliness.

A far more respectful attitude pervaded society generally in those days. People were certainly more considerate towards each other and good manners were accepted as a norm. People were expected to dress in a way that didn't offend others and to 'do as you would be done by'. Children simply didn't disrespect or disobey their parents. They were expected to 'be seen and not heard' when in company.

An attitude of respect was also extended to other figures of 'authority' in society. The teacher, the priest, the policeman and the doctor were held in high esteem by all and greatly respected. Giving back-chat to parents or to other authority figures would have been classed as unacceptable. Being insolent to teachers would probably result in a caning – at that time a perfectly legal form of punishment.

To the reader this may all sound bizarre, – 'life Jim, but not as we know it'. Having grown up during that period, the author can testify to the truth of the above description. This was how society operated in that 'golden' post war era. In the 21st Century we may not find this approach to life particularly attractive, but an important result was that more cohesive families provided the conditions that growing children needed. Families stuck together and people generally enjoyed better mental health. This created a far more balanced society compared to the one we inhabit at the moment. I hope the reader can appreciate what a different world it was in the 1950s and 1960s. The result of the social norms described above was a far gentler and more considerate society. It was a society that valued truth, honesty and morality – three words that have come under a great deal of pressure in the early 21st Century. It was a time of calm before the storm that we now find ourselves in, with all the social problems we now experience.

The Age of Majority

Were we right to bring the age of majority down to 18? This begs the question of when a young person is mature enough to act in such a way that they don't cause risk to themselves or others. The following recent findings might have some bearings on this question.

It's obvious to any parent that teenagers are more prone to take silly risks and find themselves in difficult situations than adults. It was previously held that this was because the risk avoidance centres of the brain didn't mature until some time in the 20s. In a more recent study, reported by Psychologies Today (June 9th 2015), it was discovered that teens are in fact very aware of risky situations. The problem is that they are prone to ignore risks when they feel observed by their peers. The following excerpt explains it in more detail:

First, during the adolescent period, there is an increased interest in peer relationships (Larson Richards, 1991), and susceptibility to peer influence increases during the early teen years and peaks at about age 14 (Berndt, 1979). Consistent with these readily observable changes in peer relationships, brain imaging studies have shown that several areas of the brain make adolescents more sensitive to the rewards of peer relationships than adults (Albert, Chein & Steinberg, 2013). This motivates teens to focus on their peers in decision-making situations that involve risky behavior.

Second, adolescents are more distressed than adults when excluded by peers. A brain region known as the right ventrolateral prefrontal cortex (PFC) might be important in helping people cope with negative evaluation from peers producing distress. Research shows that this brain region is used more heavily by adults when being socially excluded than by adolescents (Sebestian, et al., 2011). When teens do use this area of the brain during peer exclusion, they report lower levels of distress (Masten, et al., 2009).

During the adolescent years, however, this brain region is still developing (Blakemore & Mills, 2014), so adolescents may not be as effective at controlling distress during peer social exclusion. This likely contributes to engaging in risky behaviors to prevent being excluded by their peers.

Third, another area of the brain, the lateral prefrontal cortex (PFC), is responsible for mature self regulation and develops gradually over the adolescence period (Albert et al., 2013). In one study, early adolescents, late adolescents, and adults behaved similarly on a computerized driving task when they were by themselves (Gardner & Steinberg, 2005). However, when they were paired with two same-aged friends, clear differences emerged. Early adolescents were more likely to engage in risky driving when friends were present. Late adolescents were somewhat more risky in their driving when they were with friends. The presence of friends had no impact on adults' driving. Using the computerized driving task in conjunction with an fMRI, researchers found that, in contrast to adults, adolescents were more likely to engage in risky driving when they knew that their friends were observing them than when they were alone (Chein, Albert, O'Brien, Uckert, & Steinberg (2011). The area of the brain that was used by the adults, the PFC, helps with decision-making and self-regulation in tasks such as driving. So we have changes in *the brain during early adolescence that make teens more focused*

on the rewards of peers and

being included in peer activities. This increased focus on peers

occurs during a time when the PFC is not yet ready to assist in

mature self-regulation. These factors provide a "perfect storm"

of opportunities for risky behavior.

This article suggests that our ancestors may have had some wisdom when they set the age of majority at 21, rather than 18. Its possible that delaying the age of majority to 21 might have had the practical advantage of lowering teenagers' risk exposure.

If any parents reading this are interested to find out how to teach youngsters to be less influenced by peer pressure, then please refer to the rest of the article for the advice it offers.

CHAPTER 2

THE MODERN ATTITUDE TO SEX

Two major factors have changed our attitude to sex. Probably the most important one was the invention of the Oral Contraceptive, otherwise known as The Pill. The first oral contraceptive, Enovid, was approved by the US Food and Drug Administration (FDA) in 1960. Initially there was a great deal of objection to its use but in 1965, Planned Parenthood of Connecticut won the U.S. Supreme Court victory, Griswold v. Connecticut (Griswold) which completely rolled back state and local laws that had outlawed the use of contraception by married couples. Following further legislation in 1965, the use of 'The Pill' was soon being regarded as a passport to sexual freedom and liberation from the old taboos by married and single alike. Later the IUD, the Intra-Uterine Device, also became available as a method of contraception. This small device copper wrapped plastic device was another factor in liberating women from the fear of unwanted pregnancies.

Since then other forms of contraception have become widely available including the 'Morning After Pill'. If taken within 72 hours (3 days) and preferably within 12 hours after a contraceptive accident or unprotected sex, it can prevent pregnancy by doing one of three things: Temporarily stops the release of an egg from the ovary. Prevents fertilization. Prevents a fertilized egg from attaching to the uterus.

Great concerns have been expressed by the medical profession and by social scientists on the accidental effects of this form of contraception. In an article entitled 'The Morning-After Pill' By Wendy Wright, Carol Denner, R.N.. and Jill Stanek, R.N., they make the following comment which indicates that the MAP has increased STDs and has become a lazy form of contraception for young people who engage in :

Questions had been raised about the effect of easy access to the morning after pill on adolescents and on sexually transmitted disease (STD) rates. Notably a groundbreaking study in the United Kingdom released in April 2004, found that 'the shift towards greater promotion of emergency birth control appears to have worsened the impact on STI (sexually transmitted infection) rates since 2000.' In 2000, regulations were passed that made it easier to dispense the morning-after pill without a doctor's prescription and initiatives introduced to promote the drug to young people.

The study concludes 'it appears that some measures aimed at reducing adolescent pregnancy rates induced changes in teenage behavior that were large enough not only to negate the intended impact on pregnancy rates but to have an adverse impact on another important area of adolescent sexual health: sexually transmitted infections'.

They go on to add;

The highly touted effectiveness of the morning-after pill leaves much to be desired, with only between 75% to 89% efficacy in decreasing the naturally occurring pregnancy rate. Up to one out of four pregnancies may still occur when it is used. Easy access to the pill may make couples more likely to engage in risky sexual activity; failure of the morning-after pill would make women more susceptible to abortion.

The article also touches on the other social effects of the MAP, especially how it enabled teenagers and older couples to take a more chaotic approach to sexuality and unwanted conceptions. Instead of being a force for good, it seems that this invention has only succeeded in adding yet more chaos to an already chaotic world.

Technology

The second factor to hugely impact society's attitude to sex is the exponential growth of computer technology, especially the internet. This has enabled easy access to sexual material, i.e. pornography, chat rooms and dating sites, and the opportunities to engage in sex related activities has gone off the charts. For those with self control, this doesn't present a problem, but for the sex addict, easy access to such opportunities is akin to putting Dracula in charge of the blood bank.

Using pornography is a type of unfaithfulness in a relationship. Every time a person uses pornography with masturbation they are cheating on their wife/husband. They are directing their sexual energies in a way that detracts from their normal sexual behaviour. They may be fantasising over images that give them an unrealistic view of femininity or masculinity. It is a delusion that pushes reality out of the picture.

The ready availability of pornography on the internet poses a huge threat to the healthy sexual development of our young people. By using porn websites, youngsters learn a warped version of sex, and a warped attitude towards the opposite gender. They are often exposed to sexual imagery before they are emotionally mature enough to understand what they are doing and how they are harming themselves in the present and in the future.

Here are a few statistics that make very chilling reading:

- Every second 28,258 users are watching pornography on the internet
- Every second $3,075.64 is being spent on pornography on the internet
- Every second 372 people are typing the word "adult" into search engines
- 40 million American people regularly visit porn sites
- 35% of all internet downloads are related to pornography
- 25% of all search engine queries are related to pornography, or about 68 million search queries a day
- One third of porn viewers are women

- Search engines get 116,000 queries every day related to child pornography
- 34% of internet users have experienced unwanted exposure to pornographic content through ads, pop up ads, misdirected links or emails
- 2.5 billion emails sent or received every day contain porn
- Every 39 minutes a new pornography video is being created in the United States
- About 200,000 Americans are pornography addicts.

Youth pornography stats

- Teenagers with frequent exposure to sexual content on TV have a substantially greater likelihood of teen pregnancy; and the likelihood of teen pregnancy was twice as high when the quantity of sexual content exposure within the viewing episodes was higher.
- Pornography viewing by teens disorients them during the developmental phase when they have to learn how to handle their sexuality and when they are most vulnerable to uncertainty about their sexual beliefs and moral values

- A significant relationship also exists among teens between frequent pornography use and feelings of loneliness, including major depression
- Adolescents exposed to high levels of pornography have lower levels of sexual self-esteem

Family/Marital pornography stats

- According to National Coalition for the Protection of Children & Families, 2010, 47% of families in the United States reported that pornography is a problem in their home.
- Pornography use increases the marital infidelity rate by more than 300%
- 40 percent of "sex addicts" lose their spouses, 58 percent suffer considerable financial losses, and about a third lose their jobs
- 68% of divorce cases involve one party meeting a new paramour over the internet while 56% involve one party having an "obsessive interest" in pornographic websites

We mustn't forget mobile phone technology, since this has also provided another convenient way of accessing pornography, dating sites, etc. The ability to carry on covert relationships through the use of the mobile phone has also contributed to the instability of many relationships and the breakdown of many families.

Now the Smart Phone has made things much easier. The new App technology allows people to make assignations for casual sex, view pornography, visit chat rooms and yet another dangerous activity, sending risque photographs across the internet, the so called 'sexting'. This latter has caused a great deal of worry for parents since the opportunity for paedophiles to groom youngsters in this way has become all too easy.

The availability of the Contraceptive Pill sparked off a huge change in sexual behaviour. The 'Sexual Revolution' as it was named, turned all of the accepted rules on their heads. Women felt safe to have sex without fearing they'd become pregnant and so were more sexually available without the commitment of marriage. Men felt liberated from the danger of fathering unintended children and so began to see sex as a recreation rather than a procreational act. Sex without commitment and responsibility allowed people to ignore the taboos that had existed previously.

This has meant that sex became for many a casual form of entertainment. Instead of regarding a member of the opposite sex as a potential mate, wife/husband, mother/father of one's children, now the big question is whether a couple will 'do it' on the first date or simply have a 'one-night stand'. Whilst the use of contraception has liberated people from the old taboos, often people still fail to use contraception, resulting in unwanted pregnancies. However being resourceful people, we've now provided a way of getting rid of these without too much bother. Its interesting to note that the same organisation, Planned Parenthood, who funded research to invent and champion the use of the Contraceptive Pill have also been instrumental in making abortion legal and widely available through their network of abortion centers.

However although its possible to get an abortion quite easily, is this necessarily a healthy thing to do? The old saying is 'look before you leap'. It's too easy to make a hasty decision without understanding that there may be repercussions that could be worse than what you are trying to avoid.

Many women in fact suffer from a type of post abortion grief that can result in long term depression and feelings of guilt and shame for having killed a child. We may not live in a religious society but the Commandment 'Thou shalt not kill' has yet to be quite erased from human memory. The sex addict who indulges in 'free sex' is able to ignore these sorts of risks and consequences, but for sure there are emotional and spiritual repercussions for creating new life and destroying it with such a cavalier attitude.

One of the biggest casualties of these changes has been the institution of marriage. Marriage was the symbol of commitment between a man and a woman to conjoin in order to create a family and hopefully a dynasty. It is a statement of intention of fidelity for the rest of one's life and a commitment to support and nurture the children that are produced. It is also, for those who marry in church, a sacred promise. Its not unusual for people born in the mid 20th century to celebrate 60 or more years' of married life. This means that families become stronger. Children not only have parents, but two sets of grandparents to nurture them. Wealth in the form of inheritances, goes down the generations ensuring that children and grandchildren have more financial security.

By opting to cohabit, it could be said that couples are expressing their lack of confidence in each other as life partners and their lack of determination to maintain the relationship for their lifetimes. Sadly, for the so called Mileniels, the latest 2018 statistics are that 42% of their relationships break down.   By undermining the family, the whole society is undermined. Their children miss out on the financial and nurturing strength that an extended family provides.

Technology has also had its effects on destabilising society. We are all aware how the internet has opened up new possibilities for communications that were previously completely unforeseen, with both positive and negative effects. It is an amazing tool that helps us with our day to day living, but it also affords darker opportunities, such as readily available pornography web sites and web sites and smart phone apps offering covert ways of contacting people for casual sex. As a result of the social pressures caused by such radical changes, there has been a huge fragmentation of society creating a great deal of misery.

Broken marriages and failed relationships have caused many social wounds. Children are often raised in homes where their needs fail to be met, and so they feel isolated, rejected and unloved. Those who take such scars into their adult lives often carry a burden of emotional pain, a lack of self worth and a craving to feel loved. The quest for something to fill the emotional void thus created is often the underlying cause for addictive states of being.

Feeling lonely, rejected and unlovable is fertile ground for addictions to be formed. Maybe addictive behavior starts as a way of achieving a few moments of oblivion from a life that is full of pain or as a way of getting some relief from a feeling of loneliness or emptiness. At the bottom of all addictions is some kind of emotional need for a quick fix that promises to take away the pain, but turns out to be only a temporary solution. Typically, that quick fix has to get bigger and more intense over time in order to have the same result, and so addiction gradually grows until it becomes a new problem to add to the pre-existing ones.

CHAPTER 3.

OTHER CONTRIBUTING FACTORS

Whatever undermines society and causes families to disintegrate will inevitably give rise to an increase in addiction. We've already seen how a very stable society prior to the 1960s was subjected to some earth shaking changes in subsequent decades. These changes had the effect of rewriting the rules that had underpinned society since time immemorial including the gender stereotypes that existed until that time.

Now that women had been released from the inevitability of pregnancy by 'the pill', they started to become ambitious to have careers outside of the home. They were often frustrated by the lack of opportunity afforded to women in a male dominated society. Feminism arose in order to redress these power imbalances between the genders.

Feminism has largely succeeded in doing this, but many are now concerned that it may have gone too far and created a new set of imbalances. Aggressive feminism has set the sexes at odds with each other, so that it now seems harder for couples to agree on the ground rules for a lasting relationship. Instead of being a relationship of different but equal partners, there often seems to be a situation where couples are locked into a competition to both be the 'alpha male' in the relationship.

Men and women, right from childhood, display completely different mental, emotional and physical characteristics. Anybody who has the opportunity to work with children, or to parent them, soon notices that there is a distinct difference in the makeup of boys and girls. That old nursery rhyme 'Sugar and spice and all things nice' hints at the gentleness of the female of the species. Boys, it goes on to say, are made of 'Frogs and snails and puppy-dog's tails', hinting at a more 'abrasive' nature.

In fact its clear that from a very early age that there is a big difference between boys and girls. Boys tend to be more active because they have far higher levels of testosterone in their bodies. This growth hormone prepares them to grow taller and to be more muscular and thick set. They are also more energetic and like to play rougher games than girls.

As a result of the high levels of testosterone, the adult male is much stronger and has far more stamina on average than the adult female. They tend to be less emotionally 'labile' than women which equips them to be able to focus without distraction. Women can't compete with men in areas where strength and stamina are needed, as evidenced by the disparity between men and women's sports accomplishments.

However when it comes to emotions, girls and women are far more 'switched on'. They are more sensitive and aware of the subtleties of relationships. Traditionally these differences led to men having more active roles that demand strength and stamina whereas women tended to gravitate to roles where less strength and more dexterity or nurturing were required. Of course this is a massive generalisation, and there are always exceptions, but still can't really be disputed.

What has happened in post industrial societies is that many jobs can now be done by both genders thanks to the invention of power tools, computerised equipment, lifting gear and automation. This has opened up opportunities for women in what were previously considered male only professions. Computerisation has created many more 'unisex' job opportunities. Women have become much more powerful and thanks to Feminism, role stereotyping has been done away with in some arenas. This has undoubtedly resulted in more options for women and better career choices. Women have obtained equal status to men in society. They have overturned the old male bias and have no need to feel subservient to the stronger sex.

However Feminism also seems to have caused antagonism between the sexes. It has caused an attitude not of cooperation, but of competition. Some women have begun to believe that they don't need men in their lives. They think they can become pregnant and then raise their children alone. This mistaken philosophy fails to take into account the children's needs. Children require both parents in their lives in order to develop a balanced attitude towards the opposite sex and to learn how to interact with them. They need to have examples of both role models in order to know what is a good parent and how to be good parents. It is true that young children really need their mothers' tender loving care or preferably the same main carer at all times. However boys around the age of

7 and upwards start to need to be with their fathers more so that they can do more boisterous activities and start learning what it is to be a man.

The Feminist view of what is acceptable has changed the nature of family life for many children now being raised in all female homes. However this goes against the beliefs of child psychologists who agree pretty much universally that both genders are necessary in order to raise balanced adults.

Moreover the single parent family is not an ideal set up. When one parent is ill, having a second provides a back up. Two parents make a stronger family unit. An extended family is stronger still.

Is There an Ideal Heterosexual Relationship? I'm going to stick my neck out and say Yes. Being from a generation that believed strongly in the benefits for individuals and society of a stable family unit, I've observed that successful and long lasting marriages/partnerships have certain characteristics. An ideal relationship needs to take into account the different strengths and needs of both partners. Mutual respect is very important in forging lasting relationships. However this quality seems to be absent in many relationships.

Being physically weaker does not make a woman inferior, but many women see themselves as having to directly compete with men to prove that they are equal. They have somehow lost sight of the true strengths of being a woman. Women may not be as physically strong as men, but their strengths lie in other areas and are equally valuable in this partnership. It is by combining the male 'yang' energy with the female 'yin' energy that a harmonious partnership can be arrived at. If a couple are both trying to be the male 'yang' energy, then the result is going to be a lack of harmony in their relationship. The man may soon start to feel emasculated and alienated. This causes friction and at some stage trust is lost and resentment starts to grow leading to an eventual breakdown.

Similarly, even though the male is stronger, his strength has to be tempered with gentleness and respect for the feminine qualities and attributes. Because he is stronger it doesn't mean he has the right to bully or physically abuse his partner. If both partners display respect to each other, communicate with each other honestly without keeping secrets and try to work as a team, then the outcome is an healthy relationship.

The image of a magnet can be used as a metaphor for the attraction between the genders. We all know that similar poles repel and opposite poles attract. By competing with men, overly aggressive and combative women repel men just like magnets of similar polarities. You can try to force them together, but sooner or later they will just fall apart.

We seem to have forgotten that men are intrinsically attracted to women because of their differences, and because they have what men lack. Men are attracted to women because of their beauty and because of their characteristics that are complementary and compatible. They aren't looking for women who want to dominate them and compete with them, but rather to be able to add their special feminine abilities to the relationship. If women can overcome their lack of self worth and the illusion that they have to compete in order to gain respect, they will enjoy better relationships. If men can give their women respect without being emasculated, they too will have lasting relationships.

After having been through a period of marital stability with very low divorce rates prior to the 1970s, we have now arrived at a time when relationship breakdown seems to be the norm. Relationship breakdown often causes a great deal of pain to both parties, but the impact of separation on the children can be far reaching. When you then factor in the likelihood of a new step parent and step siblings, children's' lives can become overwhelmingly complex. The pain of separation from a parent can be multiplied by the difficulty of relating to these new family members. A whole new generation of wounded children, and thus wounded adults, has been created as a result of this fragmentation.

Recreational Drugs

Another big factor that has accelerated the breakdown of society is the 'explosion' in the use of recreational drugs. A whole generation of people from the 1970s onwards have retreated into an emotion-numbing fog of Marijuana, Ecstasy and more recently, 'legal highs' in their attempt to deaden their emotional pain. A proportion of these have gone on to take stronger drugs with more disastrous consequences on them and on society in general. It has had the effect of further weakening the bonds in society and creating yet more emotionally wounded people.

Too many young people have had their lives blighted by drug addiction which has also impacted directly on their ability to parent and cohabit. Its easy to create children, but to parent them takes at least 20 years of consistent effort. The hurt caused to the children of drug addicts has also had an impact on society and is beginning to be a major problem.

On their website the National Society for the Prevention of Cruelty to Children says:

Over the last 3 years, 25,000 contacts to the NSPCC helpline raised concerns of substance abuse near children. The number of contacts has increased by 16 per cent since 2013/14, with 8,500 people from across the UK contacting us last year. Substance misuse is a significant risk for children and often leads to neglect and abuse. Excessive alcohol consumption or use of drugs inevitably make it difficult for parents to deal with family life and often puts pressure on relationships. Children's feelings, their relationship with their parents and how they're looked after are all

affected.

The anger and sadness felt by the children of addicts taken forward into their adult lives can cause many emotional and mental problems in later years. As a result many struggle to make lasting relationships because their own parents have let them down through addiction. The more emotionally damaged adults we have in society, the more fractured society becomes and this is the cause of yet more addiction problems for the future. Sexual addiction has only recently been recognised as an official condition, however, my work as a therapist during the first decade of the millennium led me to realise that it was already affecting many people.

Universities

Although the reader may be surprised to see the above heading, in fact the sexually 'liberated' environment in our universities must be one of the most corruptive influences of young people. We send our sons and daughters off to gain a higher education, but what we aren't always aware of is the sort of culture that they will be exposed to before they are emotionally or mentally prepared.

Freshers Fair is a notorious opportunity for youngsters to be touted by the purveyors of all sorts of negative influences. This can make university a hot bed of dubious activities that their parents might not be so pleased to know they are exposed to.

CHAPTER 4
WHAT IS SEXUAL ADDICTION?

Whatever undermines the family will inevitably create wounded adults with mental health issues. In a society where everybody is looking to self medicate in order to dull their pain and fill their feelings of sadness and emptiness, its easy for people to confuse the orgasmic charge of sex as a 'cure' in the same way that drugs are used to numb emotional pain.

The warmth and intimacy of the sexual act is easily confused with something that all are seeking; to feel loved. In our craving to diminish the feeling of loneliness and isolation, sex is increasingly used as the 'drug of choice', whether it's through multiple sexual relationships or by the use of porn and masturbation.

Sex has been used as a marketing tool to sell commodities. Sex has been used to sell films, fast cars, cigarettes and a wide range of goods. According to Psychology for Marketers website, the use of sex in advertising goes back almost to the beginning of that industry.

History of sex and marketing

The fact that sex sells is not a recent invention. The earliest known use of sex in advertising dates back to 1871, when Pearl Tobacco featured a naked maiden on the package cover. In fact, the first brands to enter this trend were: saloons, tonics, and tobacco.

In 1885 W. Duke & Sons inserted sexually provocative trading cards of actresses in their packages of Duke's Cigarettes.

Then in 1970s a hair dye Clairol (by Procter&Gamble) launched its famous campaign under the ambiguous slogan: "Does she… or doesn't she? Only her hairdresser knows for sure".

When talking about sex and marketing you cannot not mention

Calvin Klein and its (in)famous advertising of jeans featuring at that

time only 16-year-old Brooke Shields. "Want to know <u>what gets</u>

<u>between me and my Calvin's</u>*? Nothing." slogan was as controversial*

as effective at driving sales. Who, in the UK, doesn't remember

the laundrette advertisement for Levi's 501 jeans?

Psychology for Marketers goes on to give their explanation of why

sex sells:

If you ever wondered whether using sex in advertising helps to sell,

here is the answer; it does.

Actually, it is one of the strongest and most effective selling tools.

The relationship between sex and marketing is a winning

combination for almost any business. However if you don't know

how to use it, you are risking putting off your potential customers.

How does using sex in advertising work?

We have what is called a lizard brain (or 'old brain'). In terms of

evolution it is the oldest part of the brain and it's responsible for

survival. It pays attention to 3 things only; food, danger and sex.

On top of your old brain, you have a mid and new brain, which take control of emotions and logical thinking. Even though our lizard

brain operates on a subconscious level (and so we are not aware of

its presence), it is continuously working, scanning environment in

search of things that could endanger you, things that you could eat

and things that you could have sex with.

This is why using sex in advertising is so powerful. Whenever a

person is exposed to a sexual message, their old brain gets

activated. And the second that happens, the old brain takes over. It

is very difficult to ignore sexual messages.

We are extremely strongly wired to react to sex. In fact, so strongly

that we will respond to messages that only imply sex. You don't

need to use pictures of fully naked models in your ads. An ankle or

a neck will work just as effectively.

We don't just see these images with our eyes; the responses to

sexual imagery go far deeper by stimulating the brain stem, (the

'lizard/old brain'). This in turn prepares us for sex by rapidly

triggering hormones within the body to ready the body for sexual

intercourse. By constantly exposing ourselves to such images, we

can induce a state of constant arousal. If we want to control this it

stands to reason that it is necessary to nip the problem at its source.

Over the years we have been gradually immured to depictions of the sexual act, even on mainstream television channels. We can now often see the sex act depicted as part of a drama on the television or in movie without particularly remarking on it. However such sexual images with their inevitable sound effects act as a profound stimulus for the viewer. Later on when one is feeling low, bored, anxious or stressed, those images may return to stimulate the sexual desire.

At one time as a result of the so called 'sexual revolution', during a very low point in the history of the movie industry, X-rated pornographic movies were on general release in the main cinemas in the UK, although thankfully this trend was short lived. It would be interesting to know how this impacted on the population and how it impacted the rates of sexual activity and addiction at the time. The fact is that the more we are exposed to sexuality in the media and in advertising, the more sexualised we become. Another concern is the early sexualisation of children. By exposing our children to sexual images, we are planting ideas prematurely in their minds.

Scientists have attempted to understand how sexual stimuli work[2], The actual mechanism is still not well understood but it is believed to be a mixture of:

   a) physiological responses via the brain stem,

   b) one's basic hormonal state and

   c) conditioning through past experiences.

It has been shown that men are the biggest consumers of visual pornography. To quote one study[1]:

'Pornographic magazines and videos directed at men are a multi-billion dollar industry while similar products directed towards women are difficult to find. It is estimated that of the 40 million adults who visit pornography websites annually, 72% are male while only 28% are female. (www.toptenREVIEWS.com, 2006). Although experimental studies support the idea that men generally respond more to sexual stimuli than women, there is not a complete understanding of this sex difference. The extent of sex differences and the exact mechanisms producing them are unclear.

The orgasm is such a powerful feeling that it is unsurprisingly highly addictive. There are similarities between sex addiction and other addictions. One study comments:

Although sex addicts crave sex for the euphoric pleasure it provides them – much like the high that drug addicts experience when they use – they also use it for other similar reasons. For them, sex has little to do with intimacy. Rather, it's an escape from painful or unpleasant emotions and a reaction to stress – in other words, it's a means of self-medicating.

A sex therapy website makes the following comment:

Just like the alcoholic, compulsive gambler, or drug addict, sex addicts are consumed with the desire to get their next fix – in spite of the risks and potential consequences. The vicious cycle of indulging in the activity, feeling guilt and remorse resolving to change, and then giving in to the craving all over again is just the same as with any other type of addiction. The similarities between the patterns of compulsive sexual behavior and other addictions are why more and more experts have come to agree that some people truly have an addiction to sex.

Finding that one is addicted to sex can be a rather unpleasant surprise. It seems odd that a purely physical act, often undertaken with little serious emotional commitment, can take such a strong hold on one's mind. With drugs we know that the body chemistry changes and then one becomes dependant on increasingly higher dosages in order to get the same buzz. Sex can have the same effects. To differentiate between normal sexuality and addictive sexuality, the term *Hypersexual Disorders* is used.

What Are Hypersexual Disorders?

These are defined as

1. Recurrent and intense sexual fantasies, sexual urges, and sexual behavior in association with excessive time consumed by sexual fantasies and urges, and by planning for and engaging in sexual behavior.

2. Repetitively engaging in these sexual fantasies, urges, and behavior in response to dysphoric mood states (e.g., anxiety, depression, boredom, irritability).

3. Repetitively engaging in sexual fantasies, urges, and behavior in response to stressful life events.

4. Repetitive but unsuccessful efforts to control or significantly reduce these sexual fantasies, urges, and behavior.
5. Repetitively engaging in sexual behavior while disregarding the risk for physical or emotional harm to self or others.

Scientific studies have concluded that the addictive power of sex is down to a mixture of causes including emotional, physical and social conditioning. One additional dimension that is rarely factored into our decisions on how we run our lives these days is the spiritual one. I'm going to talk about this in the next section.

CHAPTER 5
THE SPIRITUAL CAUSES

In the west we have become disconnected from the spiritual dimension of our own existence. Some people believe in ghosts, many visit Mediums in order to find out about the future or perhaps read their horoscopes in the magazines. Some people report having experienced Out of Body experiences or Near Death Experiences. However, the vast majority these days seem to be uninterested in such things and we are largely a secular and spiritually unaware society these days. We have felt more insulated from death and questions of the afterlife than at any other time in the last 2000 years. A lot of people wrongly equate spirituality with being religious, but these aren't the same thing at all and I'd like to try and clarify the difference.

Every person is a fusion of the physical body, the mind, the emotions and the human spirit. We are all pretty familiar with the first three, but the last item, the human spirit is harder to define in western terms. It is often wrongly equated with vivacity or hunger for life but in fact has a more specific meaning.

A student of eastern philosophies such as Yoga or Buddhism learns early on that the physical human form is surrounded and pervaded by a finer electromagnetic substance. In some eastern philosophies it's known as Chi, Ki or Prana. The totality of this electromagnetic field is known as the aura.

In fact the aura is quite a complex structure and is related to the acupuncture meridians of the Chinese system. Such a huge topic can't be described in detail here, but if you are interested to study the human spirit's anatomy, there will be references at the end of the book that you can follow up.

But how can we prove that the human spirit exists and if so, how does it affect us and what is its role in sexual addiction? I'm going to attempt to convey this, but would ask the reader to bear in mind that although this information may be new to them, it is by no means new. This knowledge, although largely ignored in the west, has existed for thousands of years in the eastern philosophies. There are many references to the human spirit in ancient texts. There aren't so many references in Western philosophies. However the Bible talks about the human spirit often because this is the bit that survives after the physical body perishes. This is the important part that we ignore at our peril.

Here is a visualisation that might help you to understand the concept better. Picture yourself in your mind's eye and then imagine stretching out around you is an electrical field a bit like a heat haze This is your aura. The aura also contains the spiritual double of everything inside your body, since it is the energy pattern of your body. When you die, part of that energy pattern lives on because it is the essence of your being which is indestructible. The rest can sometimes be seen in the form of a 'ghost' before eventually disintegrating completely.

Everything is made of energy. We are all aware that life is created in the cells by the transmission of electrons. Nerve impulses, brain waves, pain, vision etc are all ways that energy is used by the body. There are different types of energy but apart from visible light which is a very narrow part of the full energy spectrum, most of it is completely invisible. Moreover, the various energies are all around us without us realising. We have energies from the sun, from the core of the earth, radio waves from space and radio waves that we create ourselves. We are pretty much unaware of these energies but they exist all around us.

The aura is a special form of energy that surrounds the physical body. Apart from Kirlian photography, there doesn't seem to be a great deal of scientific information on this topic. However there are people who apparently can see the aura in its full multicolour glory. Although I am not one of these, I do have the ability under some circumstances to see what is called the 'Gross Aura' which resembles a heat haze around the body. I have met a number of people who can see the full aura. One of my friends is an artist and can not only see the aura, but is able to do illustrations of what she sees.

The aura contains the energy pathways known as the Meridians, As a fully trained acupuncturist, I am very familiar with these and the effects that treatment has upon them. Having worked in this profession for a decade or so, I developed the ability to feel the acupuncture points and to sense this form of energy. Sickness can start in the meridians and then percolate into the physical body causing pain and other symptoms. There is also a connection between the mind and the meridians, so depression and sadness can also be the starting point for disease. This is the way that the spirit and the mind connect with the physical body.

The spirit is affected by everything that affects your physical body, mind and emotions. If you are happy it expands and vibrates quicker, but if you are sad it shrinks and feels heavy. If you are well it expands and glows with colour but if you are sick it becomes a grey colour and may leak energy. People who have 'spiritual vision' and can see other peoples' auras are known as clairvoyants. One such healer once advised me that my aura was grey. He didn't know my health situation, but in fact it coincided with a period when I had IBS and felt very ill.

Its true that most of us can't see or feel this electrical field, but we may become aware of it though other means. We can feel the effects when we are near a person who's aura is heavy because they may make us feel heavy too. Some negative people suck energy from others and have been referred to as *energy vampires* by some authors. Other people are surrounded by very negative 'prickly' energy and this may make one feel pushed away.

Some people are so positive and loving that its easy to sense a loving field of energy around them. I recently came across some Hari Krishna monks in the streets of a local town giving out books to passers by. Their auras were pure love. If you have a favourite person in your life who loves you unconditionally and makes you feel warm and secure, this is their loving aura that you are sensing.

Spiritual Ties

When we love somebody particularly deeply we form spiritual ties that literally connect us together. This can also occur during sexual contact. I once felt spiritual ties shooting from my spiritual heart into the heart of a loved one when we hugged. I wonder if the reader has ever experienced this?

This experience convinced me of the existence of direct spirit to spirit ties. When somebody that we love dies unexpectedly, these spiritual ties may be suddenly disconnected and then we can experience a very deep sense of heart brokenness and grief. I felt this sort of grief once when my favourite pet dog died suddenly. It manifested as a pain in the centre of my chest, coinciding with my spiritual heart, also known as the Heart Chakra.

Soul Recognition

Sometimes we may meet a person that we've never met before and yet feel that we've known them forever. This is another effect of the spirit. It can be because we are members of the same 'Spirit Family' and are connected to them in the spiritual dimension. I've come across this phenomenon quite frequently. I had this experience with a lady that I met on a charity convoy to Croatia. I couldn't possibly have met her before and yet we felt like we'd known each other for ages and we are still good friends many years later.

One friend came to me in a very nervous state. He is happily married to a beautiful young wife but had met a lady with whom he felt this spiritual connection. He was deeply troubled and had a feeling that he may be with the wrong person. However when I explained the Soul Family effect to him he was reassured and went away happy. If we meet somebody from the same soul family this doesn't make us 'twin flames' as this is an erroneous idea that doesn't exist.

Another example of soul recognition occurred to me when I was working as a professional therapist. I'd been treating a lady who was pregnant because she had problems with food intolerances. A few years later I was in the play park with my grand children and came face to face with a young boy on one of the pieces of play equipment. I felt an instant recognition and yet I'd never met him before. The reason for this recognition was soon revealed as his mother came and greeted me warmly. It was none other than the lady I'd treated during her pregnancy. I had experienced a soul recognition of the little boy who'd been in her womb at the time. The reader may be thinking that this was merely a case of the young boy looking like his mother and triggering my memory, but it really wasn't like that.

I hope that the examples above have given you some insights as to how the spirit can manifest itself. Maybe you recognised some of these situations in your own life. The human spirit is real and it has a direct impact on the well being of body, mind and emotions. You will soon learn that it is necessary to tackle the roots of Sexual Addiction whether they manifest in body, mind, emotions or spirit.

I mentioned earlier that often people are put off from discussing the human spirit because they think that is a religious topic. These days there is a great deal of confusion in this area and I'd like to clarify the differences. The human spirit belongs to the individual just as one's arms and legs do. The bodily systems all use electrical energy in one form or another. The nervous system runs on electrical impulses and every single cell generates electrons in the mitochondria. However the aura is a yet finer form of electricity.

Sensing the Qi

I worked for many years as a yoga teacher and one of the warm up exercises I regularly did with my classes is a form called Chi Gung or Qigong, meaning Energy Work. It is an exercise form linked to the more well known Tai Chi.

These exercises used to really fascinate my yoga students because they allowed them to feel this spiritual energy building up between their hands. If you are reading this on an electronic copy then you can click on the following link to spend some time enjoying Chi Gung (Qigong) Exercises. You may well start to feel the energy building up in your body and especially in your hands. If you are reading a paper copy then you'll find this link at the end of the book.

These are examples of more ways of connecting to the human spirit and knowing that it exists without being able to see it. Next I'd like to talk about how the Spirit differs from religion.

Religion is mankind's attempt to communicate with the Supernatural whether it is a Shaman contacting nature spirits, or a Priest mediating between his congregation and God. People talk about religion and spirituality as being synonymous. However, for the moment I'd like you to see these two things as being quite different.

There is a crossover between the human spirit and religion, in that the human spirit is eternal and survives the death of the body. If we think of religion as our attempt to understand the eternal, then what happens to the human spirit is obviously relevant to that discussion. There is much debate as to what happens to the human spirit after we die, but this topic won't be covered in this volume.

There are many people who are spiritual, but not at all religious, just as there are religious people who have no inkling of the existence of the human spirit, focusing their attention on the Divine spirit instead. We all have a spirit even if we don't know it and even if we don't believe in it. The human spirit affects us because it is a direct link between the physical and the emotions. The more we are aware of the human spirit, the better it is because we can then factor this into our health regime.

So how does the human spirit affect one's health? Can we do things to strengthen and heal our spirit? Will this enable us to restore our health, emotions and well being? It turns out that the answer to all of the above questions is affirmative.

A healthy spirit is one that has a strong boundary around it; a bit like the rubber skin of a balloon.. This is a natural boundary that keeps us safe from negative energy in the environment. If this boundary is damaged, then it will allow the wrong sort of energy to enter into the aura. Let's use a metaphor to help visualise this image.

Imagine you are tuned to a station on your radio. While you are receiving the signal clearly, you will hear the voices or music clearly. However if there is some interference from another radio source, the sounds will be jumbled up together and start to hurt your ears.

It is the same with a damaged aura boundary. It can allow the wrong frequencies of energy to enter your spiritual space and this can cause all sorts of discomfort in any part of one's being. You may feel heavy or depressed or experience pain somewhere in your body. These are the sort of pains that we take to the doctor but they fail to find a cause; the so called *idiopathic* illnesses. Some people even hear noises or 'see' things or may become oversensitive to other peoples' emotions.

Another aspect of the human spirit is that the aura can be affected by trauma (emotional or physical) or substance abuse. Taking recreational drugs can weaken the aura boundary so that it becomes porous and allows negative energies to enter far more easily. This can give rise to schizophrenia and other mental illnesses.

CHAPTER 6
THE EMOTIONAL CURE

So if we take this information and apply it to the problem of sexual addiction, it becomes apparent that often people are predisposed to become addicted through a history of emotional problems caused by family breakdown or other traumas. Rejection and loss can affect the emotions first and then work through the spirit into the whole person. The younger this takes place, the deeper the wounds.

The broken spiritual ties that result from relationship breakdown can leave one with a deep emotional wound to the spiritual heart. It is the attempt to heal this wound by any means that leads people into addictive states including sexual addiction. The addict tries to heal his broken heart not with love, but with lust, but this is a perversion of what the spirit really needs.

For somebody who feels rejected or deserted, the real deep need is for love and reassurance. However its often impossible to get that love, or to feel that love from parents who are themselves heartbroken through relationship breakdown or loss. Or from parents who are absent through drug use or mental illness.

This can lead people to frantically seek for love in any place they can find it. A friend once confided in me that during her teenage years she became a prostitute. She later realised that it had been a desperate attempt to find love. The child of a broken marriage and a depressed mother, she had sustained a deep wound to the heart. I can however happily report that she fully recovered from this nightmare. When I met her she was a happily married lady with a stable family and a very good job. Her life had turned completely around. She's an example of somebody who recovered their life from a state of sexual addiction.

I met her during my time working for the Samaritans; she was a fellow volunteer and I often shared a shift with her. Her recovery from her past has demonstrated that people who have turned their lives around often have a deep desire to help others who are struggling. This shows that her heart had not only healed, but she had also evolved beyond the heart pain and was able to operate from a completely different level of being.

Spiritual wounding causes the aura boundary to become leaky. This can happen through extreme emotional and physical trauma such as abuse, violence, accidents or grief. A leaky aura, instead of protecting. allows negative energy to enter into the spirit. One may start to feel a bit odd at first, spacey and fuzzy headed and gradually get worse. Some people totally dissociate from fearful situations and their aura floats above their body making them feel numb and out of contact with life.

When one engages in pornography it is like opening a door into the spirit repositories and asking all of the worst energies to come in and take residence. These energies enter and latch on to the human spirit and then do their worst. That is why the longer the problem persists, the worse it gets.

Having sex with multiple partners is also very dangerous for the spirit. We may tell ourselves that 'it doesn't mean anything' or 'its just for fun' but in fact when we have sex with another person, we create spiritual chords from our spirit into theirs. These chords are more likely to run from the root chakra which is associated with sex rather than the heart. If we have created spiritual chords with a drug user or with a prostitute, then our spirit will be permanently affected by their energy. These ties will remain in perpetuity unless some positive action is taken to remove them.

Masturbation is also a very dangerous thing to engage in as it draws a particular 'Spirit of Lust' into the aura. This energy literally fixes itself onto the genitals and won't let go unless one uses particular strategies.

Curing sexual addiction is a difficult or impossible if you try to tackle it with 'western' medicine and philosophy. These are ailments of the spirit, and so it is necessary to use spiritual cures in order to bring about healing and restoration. However for those who have had a history of emotional problems, its wise to attend counselling to talk about these problems IN PARALLEL WITH using the spiritual approach.

There is another important condition for success. To effect a cure its necessary to be willing to do things differently. We tend to get stuck in behaviour patterns and many of these are 'fear based avoidance techniques'. In other words we do things out of fear because we think they will help us in some way. If these strategies haven't worked, then one has to be able to acknowledge this and be prepared to accept suggestions for new ways of being. In life we all need to be 'open and teachable' and be prepared to sometimes go out of our comfort zone as this is the only way that we ever learn and develop. By being open to new ways of doing things and new ways of living we will have a better chance of success.

Acknowledging

The very fact that you are reading this book shows that you have already acknowledged there's a problem and you want to find a solution. The starting point is acknowledging those areas of brokenness in your life.

You are probably only too aware of the emotional traumas that caused wounds to your heart. It would be a good idea to write these traumas down, without going into too much detail. As you do this, ask yourself what negative feelings and negative self beliefs you took on board as a result. Did you start to feel rejected, worthless, unlovable? These are all the sort of lies that we so easily believe.

If we've been rejected, especially in childhood, it is all too easy to blame ourselves. We start to believe that we are unlovable, and that we deserve the rejection or ill treatment that we've experienced. These feelings can be lodged at a very deep place in the spirit so healing such hurt takes something equally profound.

The next acknowledgement is that the behaviours we've engaged in order to fill the void and numb the feelings of loneliness and emptiness have had a harmful effect on us. They haven't worked, except for a brief and illusiory moment of relief, and in fact have led to an addictive situation. You have ended in a worse situation overall and this is blocking you from developing normal relationships and having a fulfilled life.

The next thing to acknowledge is that you may have done things that you regret now. The important thing to remember is that we none of us go out with the intention of making mistakes. We usually try to do what we think is best, but without guidance and experience we all too often fail. This is a fact of being human. However rather than beating ourselves up about it, we need to use these experiences positively. We need to learn the lessons that they have presented us and this is a positive outcome.

The next acknowledgement is that life/behaviour changes need to be made if we want our lives to improve. As I often say to the clients that I counsel, if we never make any changes then things will always remain the same. One will benefit the most by striving to be open and teachable. Although some of the suggestions in this book may be foreign to your normal methods of thinking, by opening your consciousness you will allow yourself to discover new ways of being.

We tend to have a sort of arrogance in the 21st century towards our ancestors. We have reaped the benefits of science and technology and have convinced ourselves that we are superior to previous generations. As a result we have often rejected the wisdom of our ancestors and looked down on them as some sort of primitives. We so easily reject the opinions of our parents as 'old fashioned' nonsense. In our arrogance we say 'I'm going to do things better than them', but 20 years down the line we may realise that we were wrong to reject their belief system and standards out of hand. When we look at the lives of our parents we may actually realise that they have been more successful because they used different life strategies. We may start to understand why they did the things their way.

I'd like to suggest that our ancestors were greater than us. Without the benefit of technology our ancestors survived and thrived. If they hadn't played their part in progressing humanity, we wouldn't have been able to build on their achievements. We stand, as the old saying goes, on the shoulders of giants.

So were we correct in rejecting their beliefs, their standards and their morals? Compared to them we are softies. We are too weak to have survived two world wars like our grand parents. We've allowed ourselves to be undermined and attacked. Our lives and our futures are under threat because we've been opened up to destructive influences that have weakened us.

The problem of Sexual Addiction is a problem of our age. Why should this be? I've already suggested that it is because we have let our standards drop. We used to live in a society where morality was important. We tend to look back and point the finger of accusation at our ancestors for being judgemental about morality.

This doesn't mean that morality was offensive, but rather that some people used others' failings as an excuse to disadvantage them. In fact morality is an important consideration in any society and it is as a direct result of living incorrectly that we are opened up to Sexual Addiction.

It is pretty obvious that this lowering of standards has affected the whole of society. The chaos that ensued has pervaded society like a fungal infection eating its way through an organism until it is so diseased that it dies.

Even a brief search on the internet shows that levels of mental health disease are progressively increasing over time. Family breakdown has led to high levels of anxiety even in quite young children. Self harming has become a common problem amongst young adults. The levels of Anorexia and Bulimia have spiralled out of control. Statistics from the States have shown that the life expectancy has dropped for the second year running. More and more people are living isolated and unhappy lives because we've forgotten how to relate to each other. We seem to have lost our way. Unhappiness and depression leave people open to addiction and sexual addiction is no exception.

In order to reverse Sexual Addiction there needs to be a two pronged attack. Firstly we have to decide to change our behaviour by avoiding the triggers that keep us sexually stimulated. This means ridding our lives of the opportunities and reminders. The second aspect of the therapy will be explained in the next chapter.

You may be wondering what we as individuals can do to restore order and tranquillity to society as a whole. How can an individual help to reverse the damaging changes that have occurred. I suppose the answer to that is that we can all only affect our own bit. The up-side of this is that if we all take better care of how we live and influence those around us, then it will have a profound effect on the whole of society. We are society and how we live as individuals and with others is vitally important.

CHAPTER 7

THE MIND-SPIRIT-BODY LINK

We've already looked at the human being in holistic terms; a meld of body, mind, emotions and spirit/aura. The problem of Sexual Addiction usually starts with some sort of emotional wound that is inflicted on young person. If this emotional wound isn't healed, it can affect the physical body as well as the spirit. During my years as a therapist/counsellor I've had an opportunity to work with many clients who suffered emotional trauma in their childhood which became physical illness later. Here is a typical case study:

Maureen's Heart Diagnosis

Maureen, a lady in her late 50s, came to counselling because of her extremely stressed and anxious state. She told me that she'd been recently diagnosed with heart problems and now she was terrified that she might be going to die prematurely. She wanted me to help her to cope with her situation and to enable her to regain a sense of composure.

During our discussions she revealed that her mother had never bonded with her. She had never experienced warm maternal love. Her mother was a demanding parent, who was never pleased and never gave praise. The daughter (my client) never felt she was good enough and this pervaded both her childhood and her adult life. She blamed herself for the lack of maternal love she received, believing it to be caused by herself in some way. She became a 'people pleaser' who's sense of inadequacy made her very nervous around other people.

In our second counselling session we spoke about why her mother had been such a difficult person. It transpired that she had been very well educated and, prior to her marriage, had been a senior manager. In those days when a woman got married and became pregnant, that event marked the immediate end of her career and she became a housewife. For this intelligent woman, being stuck in the home was a great disappointment after such a promising career. However perhaps even more damaging emotionally was that she had been very ill immediately after the birth of my client and she had failed to have that special bonding period essential to all newborns and their mothers. This lack of an opportunity to bond contributed to her inability to give my client a normal, loving childhood.

I reflected back to my client that their lack of bonding was caused by her mother's very unfortunate post birth illness and she started to understand and feel compassion for her mother. When she also considered the frustrations that her mother felt on losing her career, she then also understood why she'd found it so hard to accept the role of mother and housewife. She then had a clearer understanding that her mother and she had both been the victims of circumstances beyond their control.

This helped her to realise that she was never an 'unlovable child' and that it wasn't her fault that her mother and she had been so distant. She then started to feel very sorry for her mother and thus was able to release the hurt and the anger that had helped to damage her emotional heart and thereby the physical heart too. It was like a load had been lifted from my client. She still had problems with her health to cope with, but the burden of emotional trauma had been lifted and its likely that she would have been able to cope better with her situation.

I hope that by now you are ready to take on board the real message of this book, which is the need to have a personal revolution and renewal of the spirit, mind and emotions. It is only through doing this that one's body can be set free from sexual addiction. The real problems reside in the spirit , but they can be healed with determination and commitment. This section is divided into three sections since one needs to make physical, emotional/mental and spiritual changes if you wish to succeed.

Physical Changes

The physical changes that I am about to suggest are about the environment you inhabit. If you have sexual imagery around you or it is easily accessible, it is necessary that you take it away, destroy it or close the accounts and close the avenues that enable you to gain access.   This isn't just because sexual imagery keeps on stimulating sexual thoughts (which of course it does) but also as a statement of intention. The fact that you have done this is the first stage of your recovery. Please be creative and thorough. If it means leaving your smartphone in somebody else's custody and purchasing a simple non smart phone for the duration, so be it. If it means removing technology from your life; so be it. Having easy access to pornography or dating sites may make it easier, in a moment of weakness, to give way to strong urges, but if the means isn't available it will be harder to do that. The more obstacles you can put in your own way the better it will be. Here are some other suggestions:

- Go through your phone and erase all the contacts and apps that will be a source of temptation.
- Get yourself busy with other interests: sign up for classes, join a single-sex gym, take up a hobby that keeps you busy mentally and physically
- Reward yourself for each day when you've avoided temptation; maybe start a holiday fund or save up for something you've been wanting. When you've been 'good' put some cash in that fund.
- Fine yourself by making a donation to charity for a day when you failed to avoid temptation. It has to be enough to be painful so that it will be a disincentive. That way at least you will be benefitting somebody so you needn't feel ashamed.

The Emotional/Mental Changes

It's essential to learn how to see the opposite gender in a different light. Maybe you've been in the habit of fantasising about them and sexualising them probably, but remember that these are people, not sexual opportunities on legs. Try to stop 'undressing' them and see them as people with families and normal lives. It is really unhelpful to be in the habit of imagining having sex with people so this needs to be reined in and stopped. Such mental habits need to be actively curbed using mental discipline. If you want to get healed, this is an essential step. When you see an attractive person, imagine your mum or dad are listening into your thoughts.

How often do non addicted people think of sex? Psychology Today recently reported on the results of a survey undertaken by Dr. Terri D. Fisher, Professor of Psychology at The Ohio State University at Mansfield:

We added up the seven daily reports for each person and then divided by seven in order to get the average daily thought frequency. It was immediately apparent that both men and women were quite variable in the frequency with which they engaged in

sexual thoughts. The tally counts reported by the men ranged from

1 to 388. The variation for the women was less extreme, but still

quite large, ranging from 1 to 140. Because there was so much

variation, it makes most sense to talk about the median scores (50th

percentile), because medians are less influenced by extreme

scores. We found that the median number of sexual thoughts for

men was 18.6 and for women it was 9.9. In contrast, the average for

men was 34.2 and for women it was 18.6. Statistical tests indicated

that the number of thoughts about sex was not statistically larger

than the number of thoughts about food and sleep.

These figures represented how often people thought about sex in a

day. The results busted the urban myth that the average male

thinks about sex every 7 seconds.

It may be worth noting how often you think about sex. The way it

was done in the above study was by each participant carrying a

clicker which they used to record whenever they had a sex related

though. It might also be useful to record/note the intensity of the

feeling and decide if it's a passing thought, a desire or a strong

craving. Once you have come to realise how often and how

strongly your mind dwells on sex, its a good idea to record this somewhere. This will be your starting reference so that after a few weeks you will be able to look back and make a comparison.

As I've already stated, addiction can often be an attempt to self medicate emotional pain. It stands to reason then, that attending to our emotional problems is a very important aspect of curing sex and other addictions.

Here are some more suggestions that are strongly recommended.

- There are organisations that help with sexual addiction. You may consider joining one of these, however I would warn against getting into organisations where you meet regularly with other sex addicts unless they are 'recovered'. I'll explain the reason for this later.
- Find a 'buddy' who can give you backup when you experience strong temptation. A buddy needs to be available on the phone to give you encouragement and talk through any 'triggers' that may have pressed emotional buttons.

- It is highly recommended that you find a counsellor who can help you talk about deep seated issues. Humanistic Counselling focuses on releasing emotional baggage and so is particularly appropriate for this cure. Find a counsellor that you feel very comfortable with and can open up to.

- In addition it is very important to have emotional support while you are undergoing counselling in case you experience an emotional crisis between sessions. Counselling can cause deep seated feelings to start percolating up into one's conscious mind and it might bring painful experiences back into sharp focus. If you don't have the emotional backup then please don't start the counselling as its not safe. Wait until the conditions are right as it will be far more successful.

Forgiveness

Forgiveness is an important part of one's recovery. It could be that you are walking around with simmering anger somewhere in your conscious or subconscious mind towards a those who caused you harm in the past. It could be that you are blaming yourself for things that have gone wrong in your life. Forgiving yourself and others who have been instrumental in causing your emotional distress will help greatly to offload a great deal of emotional tension.

Being in a state of non-forgiveness means that we carry around a burden of bitterness and anger which can be the main fuel feeding addictive behaviour. Very often, those whom we are hating and not forgiving are completely oblivious to our ongoing suffering. They moved on a long time ago and for them, you and what they did to you, are just a forgotten memory, so the only one who continues to suffer is you. In this way, by holding on to non-forgiveness, we simply prolong our own suffering.

It's important to know that those who hurt us were often hurt themselves first by others. Problems can roll down the generations a bit like snowballs rolling down a mountain side. In this case it is very arguable that whatever harmful actions they did to us, it wasn't really their fault. Broken people do horrible things; its a sad fact.

Sometimes people behave badly through genetically inherited character traits such as Autism. Autism and a milder form, Aspergers, are two very common mental disorder caused by anomalies in the brain or brain chemistry. For no fault of their own, autistic people may lack the empathy that is necessary to create healthy relationships. They also have problems in interpreting normal bahaviour and reacting to it appropriately. If they happen to be parents, then it is very sad for their children who are often brought up in an atmosphere lacking in the love that they need. '

In a similar way, people often suffer from depression and other mental problems and these too will cause poor relationships and poor parenting. Other problems like illness, injury and addictions can also interfere with the parent child relationship. The following case study illustrates this sad fact:

Helen's Story

I never met Helen face to face as I only counselled her online, thanks to the wonders of the internet. Her's was a particularly sad story. She explained to me that she'd been brought up by a very dysfunctional couple.

Her father had fallen from a height when she was very young sustaining an injury which rendered him disabled. He was often in a lot of pain and this affected him deeply. His career was ended and he became deeply bitter about what had happened to him. Bitterness and anger ruled his life and he often took it out on Helen's mother. She became a very depressed person; she was often tearful and withdrawn and then was unable to show love to Helen.

Sadly young Helen grew up in that atmosphere of anger and bitterness and neither parent was able to supply her with the love and reassurance that she needed. Her father was also a very critical person and this deeply affected her self confidence because she never felt good enough.

Because of her difficult upbringing she never felt comfortable around people, even at school and tended to keep herself to herself. As a result, she had never had a relationship with anybody from the opposite sex and because of this she felt a deep sense of shame. She was so scared of revealing this to any living person because she feared that she would be judged by them. As a result she stayed single and isolated. She had a job and was able to perform it well, but whenever there was any social interaction she would make excuses and leave. She lived with her elderly mother who was the only person that she ever socialized with. Her fear of judgement and her shame was keeping her in total isolation.

Unfortunately, Helen's problems go very deep so online counselling, whilst giving her an outlet to talk about her suffering, is going to take a long time to change her deeply held self hatred and sense of shame. Counselling is effective for many clients, but for Helen's very deep trauma, a much more holistic approach is needed. The holistic approach is what I am recommending to the reader since it works on the body, mind, emotions and human spirit.

In the modern world where many relationships will break down sooner or later, step mother, step father and step-sibling relationships create huge challenges. Children can suffer enormously as another client demonstrated:

Sandra's Story

Sandra was sent for counselling by her physician because she suffered chronic depression. She'd been on antidepressants for many years, with no apparent improvement. She was reluctant to come to counselling and had only done so because of threats to withdraw her medication.

It soon became clear that her problems had started in childhood. After the death of her mother, her father married a woman who already had two children. Her step mother had apparently resented Sandra's existence from the start. She always put on an act of being a good step mother when Sandra's father was around, but when he left the home each day to go to work she changed in her attitude and treatment of my client. She became very hard and cruel towards her, whilst being kind and generous to her own children.

This left a huge burden of resentment and anger within my client. I felt that this was a huge and heavy burden that she dragged behind her wherever she went. The anger and hatred still simmered within her in spite of the fact that she was now an adult in her early 40s, and her step mother was an elderly woman suffering from dementia.

When I explained to her that her anger was causing the depression she could appreciate that this was true. However, when I asked her to find it in her heart to forgive, she was completely unable to do so. I wish that I could report a successful outcome for this client, but at the time when her 6 weeks of NHS counselling was finished, she seemed no nearer to having forgiven her step mother than when she started our sessions. I can only hope that a seed was sown during those sessions and that eventually she was able to come to the stage where she could forgive and move on.

This client was particularly bitter and the trauma was particularly deep. For most of us, once we realise that there were reasons for people acting out against us, it becomes easier to forgive them. If we realise that by holding onto anger and non forgiveness, we prolong our own suffering, then it makes sense to try to work on this problem.

How do we forgive? I've often had clients ask this question and it is a very relevant one. Where one has been deeply wounded, feelings of pain will continue to percolate up into the conscious mind, bringing back the suffering over and over again. This can make it seem as if forgiveness is impossible to achieve.

For this reason I often advise my clients to break the task of forgiveness down into two stages. The first stage is fairly easy, once we gain an adult understanding of why things went wrong. The second stage is one that can take place in its own time. Experiencing the emotions again doesn't mean you have failed to forgive; it just means that you need more time to process the emotions. This means that once you have done stage 1, you have already forgiven and that is the most important part. The two stages are as follows:

1. **Forgive 'logically'.** Knowing that you need to forgive for your own well being means its easier to take the logical decision to forgive. Say to yourself or out loud 'I declare that I have now forgiven ....for having hurt me by .... Congratulations! you have 'officially' forgiven whoever it was for doing whatever they did to you. Celebrate this landmark moment in time.

2. **Allow the emotions to heal over time**. The idea of this is that whenever hurt feelings percolate up into our conscious mind, we acknowledge them and don't try to suppress them. Write down these feelings on a piece of paper and make a ritual of safely burning it. As the paper burns, let go of the hurt with a realisation that this is healing your heart and making you stronger. If you believe in a higher power, then you can hand over the pain to that higher power for healing.

Meditation

One of the most healing things that you can do for the emotions is to learn to meditate. In my job as a yoga teacher I regularly taught meditation and can testify to the beneficial effects it had on my students.

I learned to meditate through attending a Buddhist centre in my locality. I can really recommend this to anybody who has a mind that is constantly whirring with negative thoughts towards self and others. Often we are crippled by anxiety or feelings of rejection. All of these mental states can be improved through learning to meditate.

One analogy for this is a cork bobbing on the ocean. On a calm day, the cork will gently bob up and down – this is the equivalent of us coasting through life when things are quite okay. On a stormy day the cork starts to be violently tossed around, sometimes going under through the force of the waves. This is a bit like the mind when it is buffeted by anxiety, fear, sadness and disappointment. If that cork can rise up and hover in the air above the waves, no matter what is going on below, it will remain still and untroubled. This is a metaphor for the effects of meditation, which enables us to be surrounded by the storms of life without being tossed around and harmed emotionally.

One big thing I gained through learning how to meditate was that I can now control my thoughts rather than my thoughts controlling me. I started to recognize the very negative thinking patterns that I had adopted in my life and learned how to stop them in their tracks. I then started to adopt more positive, life affirming ways of thinking. In this way I was able to grow mentally stronger and so, was less attacked by the negativity that surrounds us all. I love the mental peace that one attains through being able to Meditate and recommend anybody to seek a school of meditation.

There are many types of meditation, but the one I learned was Tibetan Buddhist style. I attended a Tibetan Buddhist Temple quite close to where I live. Tibetan Buddhism isn't pure; it is a mixture of an ancient animistic shamanistic religion called Bon that predated Buddhism arriving in that country. Buddhism was imported from Nepal and China. Wikipedia gives the following explanation, although other explanations exist.

Although Buddhist scriptures may have made their way into Tibet centuries earlier, the history of Buddhism in Tibet effectively begins in 641 CE. In that year, King Songtsen Gampo (d. ca. 650) unified Tibet through military conquest and took two Buddhist wives, Princess Bhrikuti of Nepal and Princess Wen Cheng of China. The princesses are credited with introducing their husband to Buddhism.

After a while I realised that Buddhism is not for me, but in any case, it was a great environment in which to learn to meditate. It is okay to take the best and leave the rest. One thing that I would really recommend is that if you want to find a school of meditation, do your homework first. There are many genuine schools, but as with everything, there are also ones that are cultish and somewhat dubious.

CHAPTER 8
THE GOD CURE FOR SEX ADDICTION

In addition to the above suggestions for the body and the mind/emotions, it is crucial that you address the spiritual aspect of the cure. The spirit of one who is suffering from any sort of addiction is sick and needs to be treated correctly to bring it back to a state of health. Just as my aura was grey during the time when I was suffering from IBS, the aura of one who is addicted is affected in some ways which will manifest as addiction symptoms, but it will also manifest in other ways, such as

- Insomnia
- Night terrors (apparitions, demon possession etc)
- Restless legs, ticks, involuntary movements
- Paranoia

- Compulsions (OCD etc)

- Delusions, voices, tinnitus

- Spiritual attachments

- Gender confusion

- Ideopathic diseases – these are ones that the doctor struggles
  to diagnose

There may be other symptoms; the above list is not comprehensive but hints at the far reaching effects of spiritual disease. Over the years when I was practising holistic therapies, various patients came for treatment for spiritual diseases. One of these was Julian. Here is his story:

Julian's Sexual Addiction

Julian was a self confessed sex addict and womanizer in his mid 30s. His modus operandi was to cruse the local bars looking for young, impressionable females to lure to his house. This was his 'love' nest, where he'd take advantage of the young females that he picked up in the bars.

I first met Julian at the Buddhist Temple; he was a fellow member of my meditation study group. One day he spoke to me requesting to come to my therapy rooms for some treatment. He'd explain, he said, when he got there.

We met as arranged and he explained his problem to me. He realised that he was addicted to sex and he knew that he was hosting a Spirit of Lust. If you haven't heard of 'Possession by spirits' before, then you can't have watched many horror movies! Although it seems like a fantasy that we exploit for its entertainment value, spirit attachment and a more severe form, spirit possession, are indeed realities. Julian knew that he had something attached to him that was driving his lust for multiple sexual partners.

He had realised that life was passing him by. Most of his friends were settling down and starting families, but he was stuck in a laddish time warp. He realised that what he craved for was a stable partnership so that he could do these things himself. The sexual addiction was preventing this from happening.

When I trained to be a therapist, I never envisaged that I would be acting as some sort of exorcist for spirit ridden patients. It wasn't something that appealed to me at all and so I came up with an idea that I felt would work. I told my client that if he wanted to have me treat him, he

had to show good faith by attending the local Christian church precisely twice. I had come to the understanding that the energy of a good church was very powerful and very spiritually cleansing. But would he agree? I was adamant that either he agreed to this, or I wouldn't treat him.

Thankfully Julian agreed to this condition. We arranged to meet the following Sunday at the morning service. He got there before me, and was 'received' by one of the elders of the church who took him under his wing. He was given a Bible to read from. I can still see him in my mind's eye holding the Bible open before him as if it were a bomb that was about to explode. He was like a fish out of water and I could see the perspiration forming on his troubled brow! I wasn't available the following week, but Julian dutifully attended church again.

When he came to see me for his first treatment I realised that he'd already undergone a profound change. His visits to church had indeed lifted off a lot of the negative energy from his aura. I was then able to treat the mental and emotional aspects of his sexual addiction. This included exploring the abuse that he'd suffered during his childhood from an older cousin which had traumatised him and made him feel a great deal of shame. He came for two more treatments and by the end of the third one, he already felt that he was on the road to recovery.

I lost touch with Julian when I stopped attending the Buddhist Centre, but about two years later I bumped into him, now sporting a beard, in a local store. He was arm in arm with his girlfriend and beamed at me. He explained that they'd been together for over a year. He said 'I knew that you weren't trying to convert me to Christianity!' and I confirmed that this hadn't been my intention in sending him to church. He had realised that it was an essential part of his treatment.

Although not my role to interfere in the religious beliefs of clients, it is certainly part of my role to heal their spirit. By sending Julian to church he had entered a high energy environment where negative energies just couldn't survive. The energy of a good, lively and spirit filled church is powerfully cleansing. It is a very charged environment because people go there to pray and this spiritual energy builds up and permeates the whole building. I was using this characteristic of my local church as a way of spiritually cleansing Julian – a task that I couldn't have done myself without risking my own health.

But you may be asking yourself 'cleansing what, why and how? And isn't cleansing something we do in the bathroom!'

In the same way that the physical body can pick up parasites, the spirit body is also prone to do the same. If you inhabit a clean environment the dangers of picking up parasites is slender. If, by contrast, we are walking through a tropical jungle full of species that are only too keen to get a free lunch or find a host for their offspring, then the dangers are much higher. Insects will attempt to lay eggs on your skin or parasite eggs may enter via your drinking water. Leaches will attach themselves on your legs to suck your blood or mosquitos may try to inject their eggs directly into your bloodstream while they take a 'snack'.

The spiritual body is similarly subjected to spiritual parasites. Again, a lot depends upon the environment that you are in. A spiritually clean environment is safe, but a spiritually dirty environment is much more liable to contain energy forms that can invade your aura or attach themselves somewhere to sap your energy.

Back in the 1950s, when I was a youngster, our spiritual environment in the UK was pretty healthy. After the second world war we had experienced extreme austerity, poverty even. People had been impoverished materially by the war, rationing and the very fact that being in national service wasn't very well paid. My father came back from his stint in the navy very poorly qualified for civvy street and very short of money. He and my mother had to work really hard to make up for lost time. Then my sister arrived on the scene and the finances took another knock because my mother became a home maker and housewife.

In spite of our financial poverty, we were rich in every other way.
We lived in an unpolluted area of Cheshire not too far from the
beautiful medieval city of Chester. Our neighbours and fellow
inhabitants were good people who respected each other and were
always there to help if anybody had a problem. The church was the
focal point and around it revolved the religious and social life of the
whole village. Everybody knew everybody and it was normal to
greet each other on the street or to spend time exchanging news.

For a child it was a perfect place to live. All us kids would spend the
long summer holidays and weekends playing together on the green
spaces in front of our homes or we'd gang together and play in each
others' gardens. Our parents weren't afraid of us being molested by
wierdos or being abducted because it just didn't happen in those
days. We could always run home if we needed mum and the back
door was always open because we didn't fear that somebody would
enter our house to steal from us. We didn't have a lot of stuff or
money to steal anyway so they would have been very disappointed.

The drug culture was yet to be imported into British society and for
sure we didn't have gangs of thugs with knives on the streets or

muggers ready to attack just to steal a mobile phone or handbag. Alcohol was something that was consumed in the pub, but only by people who were afflicted by some unnatural need to waste their hard earned wages in order to get drunk. Most people were happy to have a cup of tea and maybe at Christmas, push the boat out with an ale or a sherry.

From this description you will conclude, I hope, that life was very safe and we felt relaxed and secure. The community spirit was extremely strong and people had no need to be anxious or stressed. Its true that we were all broke, but that didn't matter. We were all broke together and so we didn't have feelings of inequality causing social divisions. People were gentle and respectful to each other. Mostly people were Christians and the ethos of this faith had a softening effect on the people in the area.

In such an environment, with emotionally healthy people and a very low incidence of mental illness and crime, it was a spiritually 'clean' place to be. One was highly unlikely to pick up any negative spiritual energy.

Contrast this with the way that we live these days. We live in an

time where we have a huge drug epidemic causing widespread

social problems. People drink much more than they used to do

thanks to higher incomes and cheaper alcohol. There is a much

higher incidence of mental illness due to the fracturing of society

and the high rates of divorce and relationship breakdown. Although

we are relatively much wealthier than we were in postwar Britain,

the costs of living have risen astronomically and there is a lot of

inequality in society. We are society of haves and have nots where

the wealth is being concentrated into fewer hands over time, which

is bound to create social problems.

This sort of environment is spiritually akin to the tropical jungle with

its army of parasites. Drug takers, without realising it, open their

auras up to absorb some very harsh energies that will result in them

being clogged and sick. People who are mentally disturbed,

stressed, angry or depressed, can create harsh energy around

them. Fear also creates a strong energy charge in the aura. All of

these energies that people carry around them can be transferred to

other people. You may be standing in the queue at the pharmacy

waiting to get your medications, and next to you is a drug addict who is queuing for Methadone. While you are next to the drug addict, his/her negative energy can leak out and invade your space.

Similarly, we may be on the underground commuting to work, standing in close proximity to somebody who is suffering from chronic depression. The dark energy that is clogging their aura can easily transfer over to their neighbouring passengers where it lodges and causes a wide range of physical or emotional problems for the new hosts. We may be sitting in the bus next to somebody who is filled with rage over some perceived hurt, and this angry 'thought form' can easily shoot off and collide with your aura causing a headache or pain somewhere in the body. Each of these invading energies is a type of energy parasite that can lodge in one's spirit and cause problems for an indefinite period.

In the spiritually clean environment of my village, one reason that people stayed healthy was that they had some regular spiritual input into their lives. As I mentioned earlier, the church was the hub of our community. Probably 80% of the residents attended either the Anglican or the Methodist church in the village. This meant that every Sunday we all got a spiritual clean up by being in the high energy environment of the church. We went home cleansed and ready to start the week. We probably didn't realise it, but we had done ourselves a power of good.

Church attendance has plummeted in Britain, largely due to the scientific revolution that has supplanted faith. The majority of people no longer believe in the existence of a spiritual dimension. Death, the spectre that stalked the world prior to the invention of the antibiotic and other clever drugs, isn't nearly the threat it used to be at one time. Atheism has spread like a cancer through society and as a result, most have done away with any form of spiritual input into their lives, seeing it as irrelevant.

However this was a big error for which we are all now paying. If we all get a spiritual clean up at least once a week, that makes a huge difference to the amount of negative energy that is being carried around and shared by the population. Whatever our view about religion, it is certain that going into a 'high energy environment' like a church is the best way to get the aura cleansed. Having been brought up as a Christian, which I rejected in my teens, I later began exploring other spiritualities, at different times being an

Atheist, Buddhist, Hindu, Yoga teacher and finally coming back to Christianity again. This means I've experienced life with and without spiritual input. The fact that I've gone in a full circle indicates a journey and a story.

As a youngster my father decided that the family should attend church and my sister and I should go to Sunday school every week without fail. When I hit my teenage rebellion years, it coincided with the so called Scientific Revolution and I lost any faith in Christianity that I'd had. I didn't have a great deal of genuine faith in the first place and I never really understood it much in spite of my years attending Sunday School. I was not only rebelling against the church, but principally against my father. There was no real reason for this as he'd always been a wonderful dad. I guess it was all part of the stupidity of being a teenager.

As I went through life as an atheist/humanist for the next thirty years, I gradually became more aware of the spiritual dimension of life. Getting married, giving birth, being a parent, being bereaved; all of the profound experiences of life have profound effects. We develop spiritually as we grow and learn. I became a closet spiritual seeker, trying to understand what I was experiencing and trying to find the truth.

A big turning point for me was when I found a book on spirituality in my son's bedroom. He'd been offered it in the street, taken it out of politeness, but then dropped it rather casually on his bedroom floor. Whilst tidying around I picked it up and started to browse it. Curious, I put it in the bathroom intending to read more when I had a long soak later that day. As I read the book I had a very strange experience; I felt tingling sensation going down my arms and I was sure it was coming off the book. The book was written by Srila Prabhupada, an Indian monk who had brought the Hari Krishna faith to the West in the latter half of the 20th century. I found the topic completely bizarre and yet at the same time compulsive. I self studied this faith for a few months sending for some more books from the publisher.

I had one particularly strong experience during my Hari Krishna days, that I now describe as a spiritual awakening. I was totally blissed out for a month with what I suppose was 'The Holy Spirit'. It's a feeling of total love that is unlike anything ever felt normally. I discovered that love isn't just a feeling, its also a type of energy or force. I came to believe that this is the real force that underpins every part of existence. Unfortunately this amazing feeling couldn't last forever and it gradually waned. From then on I had to find out more so that I could explain to myself the reasons for this amazing experience and hopefully regain it.

Yoga had been an interest of mine since my early 20s, but only as a method of relaxing, reducing stress and keeping my weight under control. My continued experience eventually enabled me to volunteer to teach a class in the gym I attended and eventually gave rise to a part time career that took me into the gyms and fitness centres in my area. It was more a vocation than a job because it brought me in contact with many people who needed help to cope with their stressful lives.

However as I deepened my knowledge and experience I also started to understand the spiritual side of yoga. This rich tradition is a part of the Indian Ayurvedic system; a comprehensive medicine system that works holistically. There is a great deal of information on the human spirit in the yoga tradition. It explains that as we grow from childhood into adulthood, and then into our later years, the spirit develops until we hopefully get to a stage of enlightenment. This is when the human spirit starts to be able to connect with the 'universal spirit'. We hopefully become more compassionate and spiritual, more psychic and intuitive.

Sadly, these days, fewer people will attain this state of spiritual enlightenment because most of the adult population have closed their minds to this aspect of their life. Because of this they are also more prone to experience spiritual diseases, which include mental diseases like schizophrenia, personality disorders and the subject of this book, sex addiction.

The Spiritual Jungle

Carrying on from the parasite analogy above, it is important to know which sorts of activities and environments are dangerous for the human spirit so that we can avoid them. Certain activities are more dangerous because they open up the human spirit and allow harmful energies to enter the aura. Once they have entered into the aura they start to cause pain, fatigue, heaviness, anxiety, compulsions and a wide range of psychoses. In the Bible there is a famous story about when Jesus heals the man who is possessed. He asks the spirits 'what is your name' and they answer 'Legion'. There are hundreds of spirits inside the possessed man and they come out of him and jump into a herd of pigs which run off the edge of a cliff to their deaths. The man is completely cured.

To many, that story may seem like a fantasy, but when one has been working in therapies, as I did for about 15 years, this story becomes a lot more credible. I've regularly experienced taking on a patient's disease during a treatment. They would leave my clinic pain free and I would limp home waiting for the earliest opportunity to go to church and divest myself of whatever it was that I had taken into my aura.

A school friend of my son's unfortunately got involved in taking drugs in his early teens. Sadly he became Schizophrenic and we'd often see him ambling along the road talking to himself. I can't prove this, but I always had a strong feeling that he was in fact spiritually possessed. People with Multiple Personality Disorder are also probably hosting multiple spirits, again I can't prove that but strongly suspect it.

Another danger area where one can become spiritually contaminated is anything to do with the sex industry. Many prostitutes are infested with Spirits of Lust so that when they have sex with a customer, these can transfer onto the new host to cause sexual obsessions and other problems. Similarly, pornographic web sites, strip joints, pole dancing clubs and anywhere sex is exploited for money can become infested with harsh energies that will latch onto the aura and be taken away by their customers.

Places where drugs are used or dealt in become charged with negative energy, as do the people who frequent these places. Drugs, illegal and some legal ones too, can damage the aura and make the aura boundary weak, making it more likely that spirits will invade. Read about the experience of one of my clients':

Matt's Story

Matt was brought by his father, for a consultation. He didn't warn me ahead of time what the problem was so I was taken by surprise.

Matt had been taking various recreational drugs for some time but the family had started to get really concerned when he told them that he was having night terrors. He was waking up in the night feeling ghostly hands around his neck squeezing until he couldn't breathe.

He came to see me under duress so its not surprising that he only came the once. He wasn't willing to open up because his father was in the same room. He seemed nervous and somewhat paranoid and this was probably a manifestation of the spirit, not wanting to reveal itself or be attacked. Sadly this was early on in my career and I wasn't so aware back then about the spiritual causes of disease. By the end of my career I'd come to the conclusion that the vast majority of my patients had spiritual problems.

This case, and others, convinced me that drugs really open up the aura to receive very harsh spiritual energies. One teacher of spiritual therapy was adamant that indulging in recreational drugs opens up satanic portals that invite harmful spirits into the world.

Satanism, Witchcraft, Wiccan and Occultism

A really good way (that I would never recommend) to invite bad spiritual energy into your life is to engage in anything to do with the occult or witchcraft in any of its guises. To do this is to open up the flood gates and soon bad health and mental problems will start to manifest.

We live in a strange time when right and wrong have become blurred thanks to a corrosive degree of Political Correctness combined with a total ignorance of the difference between good and evil. I became aware that some of the so-called acceptable faces of occultism, such as Wiccan, are merely the sanitised end of a spectrum that can lead people into the much darker and more dangerous areas of witchcraft and satanism. The following is just one of the many experiences I had of dealing with people who became seriously affected by their dabblings in the occult.

Jess's Story

I spent some years involved in Reiki and found myself teaching a course at the local technical college. Reiki is based on a belief in

God and that his power can be harnessed through healing intent. This is the way I taught Reiki, as a God given gift.

I noticed that many people in the class were wearing symbols of witchcraft and I spoke to the whole group one evening about needing to be working in line with the ethos of Reiki, i.e. that the healing was of God. As a Christian I had read in the Old Testament how God had shown his dislike for anything to do with witchcraft and so I recommended people not to wear these symbols during the class, and if possible to think about not wearing them again as to do so was, I believe, endangering their health. I quoted them many passages in the Bible that were relevant.

I was pleased that most of the students listened to what I requested and cooperated with me. I insisted that those who wouldn't cooperate should consider leaving the group, and a few feathers were very ruffled. Jess continued to attend the course without her usual Wiccan five pointed star so I continued to teach the group. I was never quite happy with the energy of the class however, and couldn't put my finger on what was happening. After the class finished one day, Jess asked if she could come for some treatment at my clinic so I made an appointment for her to visit.

She explained that she had a history of mental problems. I took some background information as usual, doing a fairly in depth case history. She came for 5 sessions and then the 6th one was at her home. As soon as I entered her house I was shocked. On every wall was an image of darkness or witchcraft. There were statues of ghosts, witches and other dark beings. The penny started to drop. On questioning Jess about this she revealed that her whole family were into the occult. I advised her that until she banished these images from her home and ceased from the occultic practices, she would probably always be dogged by mental illness since these were acting as doorways for harmful energy to enter her spirit. During this period Jess had to spend some time in the local mental hospital but after she was released she contacted me again.

The next time I saw her she came to my clinic. Winter was definitely behind us and the day had turned out warmer than expected. Jess peeled off her sweater in my treatment room to reveal the five pointed star, which she'd never stopped wearing but had simply secreted under her sweater. I expressed my disappointment that she'd totally ignored that I'd asked her not to wear it and the reasons why I'd done so. Her dishonesty had impeded the treatment from working and caused her to remain mentally ill. I had to explain that therapy is a relationship of trust. If I couldn't trust her to follow the advice that I was giving, then it was pointless to continue to work with her. This was the last time I saw her but before she left I recommended that she threw the five pointed star into the river for the sake of her future well being.

In case you are puzzled by my dislike of the five pointed star symbol, I just need to clarify that it is a symbol of witchcraft, also known as the pentagram or pentangle. It is used in witchcraft ceremonies, some of which can be very dark indeed involving blood sacrifices and other unwise activities. If it is worn with this intent is connects the wearer to a very dark realm of destructive energies, which is why I believe Jess wasn't able to heal in spite of my best efforts. I never charged Jess for a single minute of my time, knowing that she was broke, so it was doubly disappointing that she'd failed to be honest with me.

Other occultic activities have the same underlying problem of connecting the participant with the dark energies that are so harmful to our health. This would include any form of witchcraft, satanism, spell making, voodoo, tarot card reading and wizardry.

Geoff's Story

I'm going to relate the story of Geoff who owned the 'Majik 'shop in my town. This was a place that I entered gingerly. The front of the shop was full of crystals, incense sticks and other fairly innocent stuff, but at the back he had a bookshelf crammed with books on witchcraft. One day I was in there when he came over to chat. He told me that he was a Warlock and that he regularly held covens. He was quite proud of this involvement. After that I steered clear of his shop. One day when I was in that part of town I noticed that the shop had closed. A poster on the window announced that this was due to the proprietor's illness. After a while the contents of the shop were removed and it became a restaurant.

I bumped into Geoff several months later and he explained that he'd been suffering from a mysterious illness that wiped out his energy totally and had him laid on his back for a few months unable to do anything for himself. Eventually he'd started to feel better and was now working as a delivery driver. I strongly suspect that it was his involvement in wizardry that was the real cause of the mystery illness.

Generational Curses

Often illnesses are described as 'genetic' because they run in families. Whilst this is true, there are other things that seem to run in families like depression, alcoholism, divorce, violence and other destructive character traits. The following case study illustrates the experience of another client,.

Edwina's Story

Edwina came on the recommendation of another client. She was suffering from food intolerances and digestive problems which I was able to treat successfully. However she also mentioned a disturbing tendency in her family for everybody to be very bad tempered with each other and to fall out which seemed to affect every generation. Her family was so broken by this tendency to quarrel and hold grudges against each other that it made any sort of family get together impossible, which was distressing for her children who wanted to see their cousins and other relatives. It became even more apparent at times like Christmas when other families were getting together and they were unable to.

I intuited that there was a generational curse on the family. Cursing used to be a common tool employed by bitter people to wreak revenge on their enemies. This goes way back into ancient history as archaeologists have found lead sheets in old Roman wells bearing curses inscribed on them. Maybe this was the origin of the idea of a ´wishing well`.

A generational curse is one that is placed on a person and all of their descendants. There are ways of clearing generational curses but I'm not going to talk about this here as its quite involved. However it might be worth exploring this as a possibility on the internet if your family seems to be dogged by such inter generational problems.

The above examples have, hopefully, given you an appreciation of the importance of spiritual health and how easy it is for it to become compromised. It has been rightly said that we are engaged in a spiritual battle these days. Our grand parents would be horrified to see the mess that we have got ourselves into through giving up on the only spiritual protection we had. They realised all to clearly how a spiritual health regime is as important, or maybe more important than any other type,

I'm going to list some of the spiritual methods for curing sexual addiction. I asked you in an earlier chapter to be open and teachable and to be ready to do things differently. Adopting new ideas and ways of behaving are crucial to effecting a change. Remember that unless you make changes in your life, it will always remain the same and the addictions will continue to ruin your life.

Here is the information you need. It's down to you now!

- Start going to church on Sundays. It helps if you can find a church where you feel at home. If you are new to these things then possibly an evangelical church will suit you as they are generally lively places with the bonus of good music and good socials

- If all your friends are into drugs, porn, sex and alcohol, then find some new friends. If you keep hanging out with the same people you'll never get free of the addictions because they will keep dragging you back.

- Look for spiritual and wholesome friends. A church is a good place to start and often has a youth group if you prefer to hang out with the younger guys.

- Avoid hanging out in the 'spiritual jungle' because this is a source of 'infection' with harsh energies that will keep your addiction going. Stay away from night clubs, drug dens; anywhere where sex and drugs are sold or used.

- Find new healthy pastimes that will make a positive difference in your life. Join hobby groups that will make you stronger and teach you new things.

- Get a Bible and sleep with it (wrapped in a towel) between your legs! I know this sounds weird, but the Spirit of Lust can be attached to the genitals and one way to detach it is to use the Holy Book.

- Find your nearest Catholic church and take an empty spray bottle with you to fill with Holy Water. There is always a dispenser or stoop available in the church for this purpose. This stuff is very useful in the battle against bad energies. It is free and nobody will stop you from taking it even if you don't attend the church normally. Spray yourself, spray your home and spray your possessions once or twice a week initially to help banish negativity from your home.

- Read the Bible – even if you don't understand it or believe it. The dark spirits do understand it and will flee from it. Read it before sleeping at night as this will help to weaken the spirits of lust and give you a better night's sleep.

- Have people at the church to pray over you. If you approach the pastor he will get a group of intercessors to pray over you. This is best done right after the communion service when the Holy Spirit is very much present.

- Have some acupuncture treatments. If you tell the acupuncturist honestly why you are attending for treatment, they will select special points that are known for clearing negative energies that cause addiction and other neuroses and psychoses.

- Tell the spirits that are invading your aura to get away from you 'In the Name of Jesus' never to return, as they no longer have any rights to be there. Their time is up, just like Legion who was banished into the pigs.

- Ask for the Spirit of Peace to fill your aura up to the brim so there's no room for anything else.

- Have positive images of spiritual subjects in your home as these will state your intent and remind you to keep up the attack.

- Ask your pastor to arrange for you to see an Exorcist. Yes, they still do exist. There are some big meetings in big churches organised for this very purpose. One well known place in London is Holy Trinity Church in Brompton. They have a good reputation for expertise in getting people sorted out and back on the right track.

- If you have a bad experience and feel you are being compromised by others, you can always use this spiritual first aid tip to cleanse your aura: Salt is very cleansing (hence the old superstition about throwing salt over the shoulder to deter the devil) and can be used in many ways. One quick fix is to have a deep bath laced with salt. Any salt will do, even the cheapest one from the supermarket. You can also use salt as a scrub if you prefer to shower.

- Bless your salt: Say this quick blessing over your salt to give it extra power

In the name of the Creator God, I bless this salt (Make the sign of the cross over it) and cast out all demons from it so that it becomes a holy medicine for body, mind, soul and spirit. May all evil spirits flee from wherever this salt is used.

- You can cleanse an area with blessed salt. Sprinkle it on and then vacuum it off. It's a sort of spiritual 'Shake and Vac' that you can use in your home wherever you feel there's a build up of bad energy.

- Have nothing whatsoever to do with witchcraft, wiccan, satanism or any dark occultic or mediumistic practices (e.g. Tarot, fortune telling, spell making). These are like putting a flag up over your head saying 'come and attack me for free'. If you have had dealings with any of these, go to a church somewhere and prayerfully declare to God that you have given up all contacts with these organisations for ever and ask to be forgiven. These practices are and always have been a kind of spiritual death. In the Bible they are the source of all the disasters that befell the nation of Israel.

CHAPTER 9

POST SCRIPT

I do hope that the information in this book will be helpful. Following the principles outlined above will help you to strengthen your body, mind, emotions and of course, the all important spirit.

- By healing the emotions through counselling and forgiveness, you will become mentally and emotionally stronger.

- Meditation can help you to stay calm while the world around you is turbulent.

- By staying out of the spiritual jungle and inhabiting a spiritually clean environment you will be safe from back sliding.

- By having some regular spiritual input into your life you will ensure that things continue to improve in every sphere of your existence. OK you may lose 'friends' initially, but you will make new ones that are more conducive to a healthy future.

It may take time for you to get over your sex addiction and to get back to enjoyment of a normal attitude to sex where you are in control. It is also possible to have a miracle cure if you are wholehearted in following the above regimes, but normally it takes time for the various cures to take full effect. Remember that it probably took years for you to become addicted so be patient in undoing the damage.

Please don't be disheartened if it takes longer than you want it to, as you will get there. Every journey begins with the first step and that is the important one. The sooner you take the first step, the sooner you will arrive at the final destination. Decide today to make the first change and then every week, or oftener if possible, make another change. Maybe the most important change is to find a good church as soon as you can.

Keep a diary of how you feel and then you'll be able to look back and make valid comparisons. You will see a steady improvement in your condition. When I treat a client I always keep a really good record of how they were on that first meeting. One of the reasons for this is that after a while, when the symptoms have disappeared, patients tend to forget they ever had them. I'm able to remind them how things were before treatment started. They are often totally amazed by the changes that have occurred. You too will be able to

see a big change.

Thank you for reading this book. Well done for being open,

teachable and willing to incorporate new ways of being into your life.

This will create huge dividends for you now and in the future.

REFERENCES

Rise in drug and alcohol related reports, NSPCC News February 2017
https://www.nspcc.org.uk/what-we-do/news-opinion/children-of-alcoholics-week/

The history of the contraceptive pill
https://www.plannedparenthood.org/files/1514/3518/7100/Pill_History_FactSheet.pdf

How often do normal, unaddicted people think of sex? Psychology Today Blog, Brian Mustanski Ph.D., The Sexual Continuum. 6th December 2011
https://www.psychologytoday.com/blog/the-sexual-continuum/201112/how-often-do-men-and-women-think-about-sex

The History of Sex and Marketing
http://psychologyformarketers.com/sex-and-marketing/

Why Are Teen Brains Designed for Risk-taking?
By Nina S. Mounts, Ph.D., guest contributor

https://www.psychologytoday.com/blog/the-wide-wide-world-psychology/201506/why-are-teen-brains-designed-risk-taking

Chi Gung Exercise Video
https://www.youtube.com/watch?v=EaEZVfhn07o

Article on the Social Effects of the Morning After Pill
https://concernedwomen.org/images/content/mapalec.pdf

Pornography statistics
https://www.webroot.com/gb/en/home/resources/tips/digital-family-life/internet-pornography-by-the-numbers

Information on the Aura
https://www.youtube.com/watch?v=vfPnVFam-ls

Made in United States
Orlando, FL
24 August 2023

36388239R00071